The

LITTLE BOOK OF

KAMA SUTRA

D1313448

THE LITTLE BOOK OF KAMA SUTRA

Copyright © Summersdale Publishers Ltd, 2015

Research by Elanor Clarke

An Hachette UK Company
www.hachette.co.uk

Summersdale Publishers Ltd
Part of Octopus Publishing Group Limited
Carmelite House
50 Victoria Embankment
LONDON
EC4Y 0DZ
UK

www.summersdale.com

Printed and bound in Malta

ISBN: 978-1-84953-778-0

Substantial discounts on bulk quantities of Summersdale books are available to corporations, professional associations and other organisations. For details contact general enquiries: telephone: +44 (0) 1243 771107, or email: enquiries@summersdale.com

The —
LITTLE BOOK OF
KAMA SUTRA

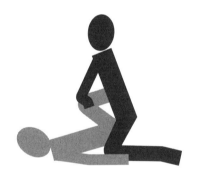

Sadie Cayman

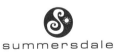

Disclaimer

Summersdale Publishers cannot be held responsible for any injuries or breakages that may occur when following the advice in this book. Always check on your partner's well-being when trying new positions, and please enjoy yourself carefully!

Contents

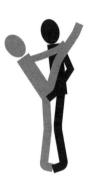

Introduction

The *Kama Sutra* is an ancient Indian text, which has been reproduced and reimagined many times over the years and provides insights into having a happy, fulfilled life with your partner. The main reason it is known in the West is for its depictions of varied sexual positions, for a satisfying sex life. While this little book can't hope to reproduce all these teachings, we've hand-picked some of the best positions and let you know how they're done, when's best to try them, and how easy or tricky they are. We have used the terms 'active' and 'passive' throughout, to show who is 'giving' and who is 'receiving' in each position. This does not necessarily show who, if anyone, is being penetrated – simply the person who is actively engaged. In nearly all of these positions, frottage (rubbing together) can be substituted for penetration and still be enjoyed by both partners!

We hope this book will prove to be informative and fun for you and your special someone. Enjoy!

P.S. Flick through the pages for a practical demonstration of one of my favourite positions, The Plough.

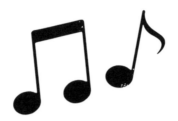

THE SEXUAL EMBRACE CAN ONLY BE COMPARED WITH MUSIC AND WITH PRAYER.

MARCUS AURELIUS

Chapter 1
KISSING

GREAT SEX ISN'T ALL ABOUT THE
ACT OF PENETRATION; THE BUILD-UP IS
IMPORTANT, TOO! ONE OF THE BEST WAYS
TO BUILD PASSION BEFORE THE 'MAIN
EVENT' IS SENSUAL KISSING, AND THIS
SECTION GIVES YOU A SMALL SELECTION
OF THE MANY WAYS THE *KAMA SUTRA*
SUGGESTS YOU ENJOY YOUR
PARTNER'S LIPS.

The
BENT KISS

PASSION:

DRAMA:

This is when each partner bends their head to the side, and moves in for the kiss. It is often depicted with the passive partner leaning backwards, while the active partner leans over them, holding them close. A 'classic' kiss, often seen at the romantic climax of films, this is popular among couples and can build great passion.

The
TURNED KISS

PASSION: ❤❤❤🤍🤍

ROMANCE: ❤❤❤❤🤍

Like the bent kiss, this one is also a classic. When the active partner takes the passive partner's chin in their hand, and turns their partner's face towards them for a kiss, this is the turned kiss. The active partner takes the lead, which adds a touch of passion to the moment. The other partner may have turned away to be coy or playful, and this kiss is a way of saying: time for the next game.

The
KISS THAT KINDLES LOVE

EFFORT:

SEXINESS:

This one is a kiss for the partner who is usually passive. When your partner is sleeping, and you feel that need for them building, using a slow, seductive kiss to wake them, ready for gentle lovemaking, is called the kiss that kindles love. Starting gently, this kiss can turn into something more passionate as your partner awakens to the world, and to you.

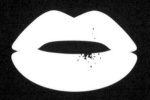

A KISS IS A LOVELY TRICK DESIGNED BY NATURE TO STOP SPEECH WHEN WORDS BECOME SUPERFLUOUS.

INGRID BERGMAN

The
KISS THAT
TURNS AWAY

COMPASSION: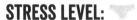

STRESS LEVEL:

This kiss is to help your partner forget about their worries, and bring their attention to you, and your relationship. When they are worrying about work, distracted, or perhaps even arguing, a gentle kiss that gradually becomes more intense will help move their attention away from the negative and back to the happiness of your embrace.

The
DEMONSTRATIVE
KISS

SUGGESTIVENESS:

DEVOTION:

This kiss is one for either in public or in private, to show your desire for your partner. Indeed, this sort of kiss doesn't even have to include both partners directly. These kisses are a visual way to say 'I want you', sometimes within a crowded room. One partner could, for example, kiss their finger whilst looking the other in the eyes. When alone, kissing your partner softly on their thigh is a good example of the demonstrative kiss.

Chapter 2

ORAL PLEASURES

ORAL SEX IS, FOR MANY, A KEY PART OF SEXUAL UNION. IT CAN BE PART OF THE BUILD-UP, OR CAN FORM THE MAIN EVENT. THE ANCIENT *KAMA SUTRA* DID NOT PUT MUCH STOCK IN ORAL SEX, VIEWING IT AS THE WORK OF EUNUCHS OR CONCUBINES, BUT THE WORLD HAS MOVED ON SINCE THEN, AND MANY REIMAGININGS OF THE *KAMA SUTRA* HAVE MOVED THEIR FOCUS TO THE INTIMATE PLEASURE ORAL SEX CAN PROVIDE. A FEW OF THE BEST POSITIONS FOR PLEASURING EACH OTHER ORALLY ARE GIVEN IN THIS SECTION.

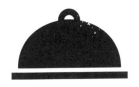

SEX IS AS IMPORTANT AS EATING OR DRINKING, AND WE OUGHT TO ALLOW THE ONE APPETITE TO BE SATISFIED WITH AS LITTLE RESTRAINT OR FALSE MODESTY AS THE OTHER.

MARQUIS DE SADE

SOLO FELLATIO

EROTICISM: 🩲 🩲 🩲 🩲 🩲

INTIMACY: 🩲 🩲 🩲 🩲 🩲

If your partner is male, there might be times when you just want to pleasure them, and enjoy the process. According to the *Kama Sutra*, the act of fellatio should be performed in several stages, gradually progressing: starting with a gentle touch of the lips, and moving on to kissing, stroking and pressing your body against your partner's intimate zone before moving in for full oral penetration. A gentle approach should be used, making it more intense if you and your partner wish to.

Don't take his penis into your mouth all at once –
alternate some long strokes of your tongue up his shaft
with shorter sweeps around the head of his penis before
taking him fully into the exhilarating heat of your mouth.
Pay attention to the opening of the urethra, run your
tongue around where the head meets the shaft, and don't
forget his balls; experiment with licking or lightly sucking
and see what gets the best response.

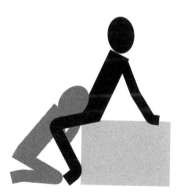

SOLO CUNNILINGUS

EROTICISM: ▼ ▼ ▼ ▼ ▼

INTIMACY: ▼ ▼ ▼ ▼ ▼

Just as with solo fellatio, if your partner is female, there might be times when you just want to give them pleasure, and enjoy doing it. According to the *Kama Sutra*, the way of kissing a woman's *yoni* (vagina) should already be known, through having kissed the mouth. This is a good place to start from, but certainly not the whole story! As with fellatio, begin gently, with kisses and caresses. Use your mouth to explore the whole of her intimate area, not just the clitoris. Some women enjoy penetration with the tongue, too. Try different levels of pressure with your tongue and lips, and find out what your partner enjoys.

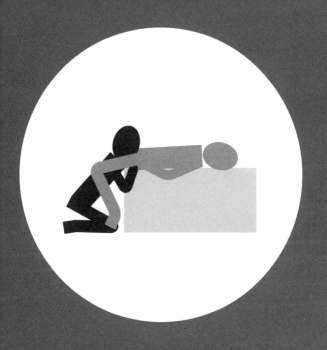

CLASSIC '69'

TWO-WAY PLEASURE:

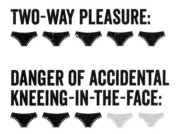

DANGER OF ACCIDENTAL KNEEING-IN-THE-FACE:

Once you've mastered the solo basics, the natural progression is to enjoy oral sex together. The most commonly known way to do this is the classic '69', named for the shape the two lovers make when they are in this position. In the *Kama Sutra*, this is referred to as 'congress of a crow'.

For a 69, one partner lies on their back, with the other on top, 'top to tail', so the bottom partner's head is in line with their partner's intimate region, and vice versa. Then, it's just a question of using the skills you've practised in solo oral sex. For many, the 69 and its related positions are a great way to have full-body intimacy with a partner, and can lead to simultaneous orgasm.

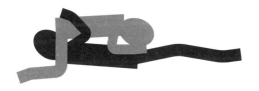

SIDE '69'

EXERTION: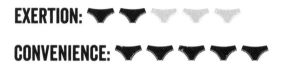

CONVENIENCE:

Like the classic, this is a simple 69 position, but rather than being one on top of the other, each partner can lie on their side in a comfortable position, with their face nuzzled between their partner's legs. This is perfect for slow, lazy sex, when you want maximum enjoyment with minimum exertion.

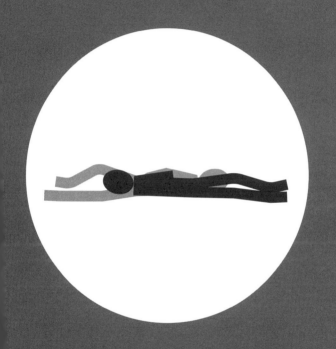

DOGGY STYLE

STIMULATION: ▼ ▼ ▼ ▼ ▽

ROMANCE: ▼ ▼ ▽ ▽ ▽

Although more commonly known as a penetrative sex position, the doggy style position can be put to great use for oral sex. One partner goes on to all fours, and the other kneels behind them, giving pleasure that way (either vaginally or anally for a female partner, anally for a male). If that's not what you fancy, then the giving partner can lie with their head below the receiving partner's intimate region, and can tease and please them from below.

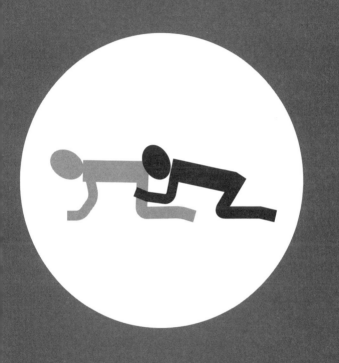

The
LAP OF LUXURY

DIFFICULTY:

PLEASURE:

This is pure laziness for the partner receiving oral pleasure. Using a favourite chair or the sofa, the passive partner sits back comfortably, while the active partner kneels in front of them, and pleasures them. The passive partner can use their hands to guide the giver, talk to them, telling them what they want, or they can just sit back, relax and enjoy the ride.

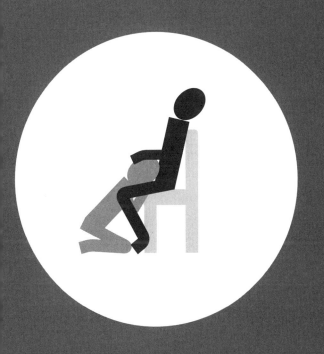

The
FACE SIT

PLAYFULNESS: 🩲 🩲 🩲 🩲 🩲

TANTALISATION: 🩲 🩲 🩲 🩲 🩲

In this position, the receiver becomes the active partner. The giver lies on the bed (or floor, sofa, etc.) with their head supported by pillows. The receiving partner then kneels over the giver's face, and gently lowers themselves down until the giver can provide oral pleasure. The giver can support the receiver by holding their hips or bottom, and the receiver can lean their hands on the wall or bed frame for extra support, if needed. This position is ideal for teasing, particularly if the giver really enjoys the part they play – the receiver can move themselves just out of reach, leaving the giver wanting more, and heightening the sense of play.

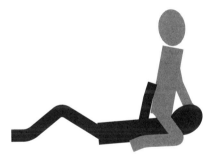

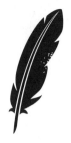

I WRITE ABOUT SEX BECAUSE OFTEN IT FEELS LIKE THE MOST IMPORTANT THING IN THE WORLD.

JEANETTE WINTERSON

Chapter 3
SUPINE POSITIONS

HERE, WE WILL LOOK AT SOME OF THE
EXCITING POSITIONS THE *KAMA SUTRA*
RECOMMENDS FOR COUPLES LYING DOWN,
AS WELL AS SOME MORE MODERN TAKES
ON THE ANCIENT TEACHINGS. THESE ARE
ALL FAIRLY SIMPLE POSITIONS, BUT THEY
OFFER AMAZING INTIMACY AND PLEASURE.

BANDOLEER

FLEXIBILITY:

PLEASURE:

This position allows for deep penetration, whilst being comfortable and supported. It is ideal for slow, lazy fun.

Start with the passive partner on their back, with their head supported by a comfy pillow. The active partner should kneel in front of them, close enough for the lucky passive person to rest their feet on their partner's chest. The passive partner can rest their thighs and bottom on the active's lap and thighs, or, if this is not comfortable, they can be supported by fluffy pillows under the small of their back. The active partner can then slowly enter, gradually building to deeper, harder penetration. For a passive partner feeling dextrous, additional pleasure can be given with manual stimulation.

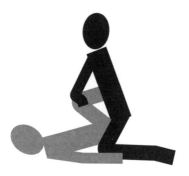

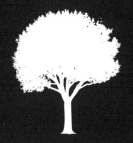

SEX LIES AT THE ROOT OF
LIFE, AND WE CAN NEVER
LEARN TO REVERENCE LIFE
UNTIL WE KNOW HOW TO
UNDERSTAND SEX.

HAVELOCK ELLIS

The
GLOWING TRIANGLE

EXERTION: ▼ ▼ ▼ ▽ ▽

CLOSENESS: ▼ ▼ ▼ ▼ ▽

This position is based, roughly, on the missionary position, where the passive partner lies on their back, and the active one climbs on top, and does all the 'work'. In this version, however, things are a little different. The partner on their back is actually the more active one.

The active partner lies on their back, with their hips
tilted upwards, ready for penetration. They can be
supported by a pillow, if this is more comfortable. The
passive partner then gets on to all fours, and enters their
partner, who then, holding on to the passive partner's
back or shoulders for support, uses the action of their
hips, back and forth, to achieve deeper penetration
(doing all the 'work'!).

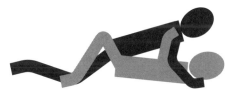

NIRVANA

SENSUALITY:

STIMULATION:

This position works best with a female passive partner, as it allows for extra clitoral stimulation, which can make orgasm faster and more intense.

The passive partner lies on their back, with their hands raised up, holding on to the headboard or bedposts. They keep their legs closed. The active partner then climbs on top, their legs spread, and penetrates their partner. The passive partner's pressed-together thighs heighten the penetrative sensation, as well as giving additional clitoral stimulation to a female partner.

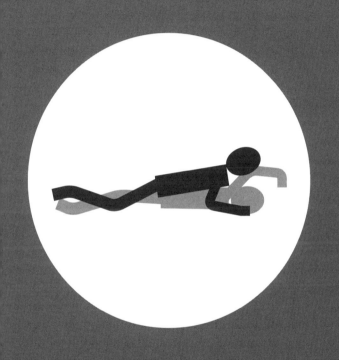

The
SPLITTING BAMBOO

FLEXIBILITY: ▼ ▼ ▼ ▼ ▼

SATISFACTION: ▼ ▼ ▼ ▼ ▼

Don't let the word 'splitting' put you off this one! It is an easy-to-do position, and great for slow, lazy sex.

To split the bamboo, the passive partner lies on their back, with one leg slightly bent. The active partner straddles this leg, then the passive partner lifts their other leg and drapes it over the active partner's shoulder, so that their legs form a scissor-like shape. A slow, sliding rhythm can be built, and the passive partner can reach down and help things along with a little manual stimulation.

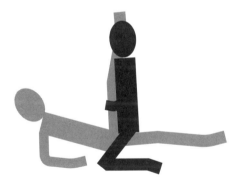

The
CURLED ANGEL

FLEXIBILITY: ▼ ▽ ▽ ▽ ▽

COMFORT: ▼ ▼ ▼ ▼ ▽

If you've ever heard the phrase 'spooning leads to forking', this position is proof.

The partner who will be penetrated curls up, and the penetrating partner curls behind them, spooning them. Penetration from this angle is soft and easy – perfect for a lazy Sunday morning – and the active partner can reach round to please the passive partner with their hand, too.

This position is often favoured by pregnant women, as it is gentler and avoids squashing the baby bump.

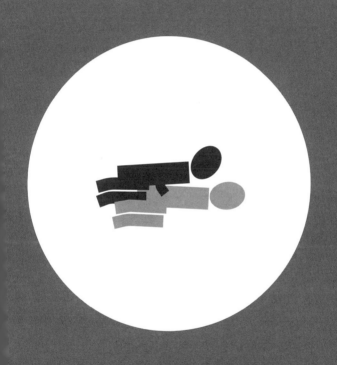

The
CLIP

SEXINESS: ▼ ▼ ▼ ▼ ▽

STIMULATION: ▼ ▼ ▼ ▼ ▼

In this relatively simple position, it is the partner being penetrated who is most active.

The passive partner lies on their back, legs closed. The active partner then straddles them, allowing for penetration, and leans back, using their hands for support. Once in position, the active partner uses a sliding movement to build rhythm, while the passive partner can reach out to stroke their skin, or give them additional pleasure using their hand.

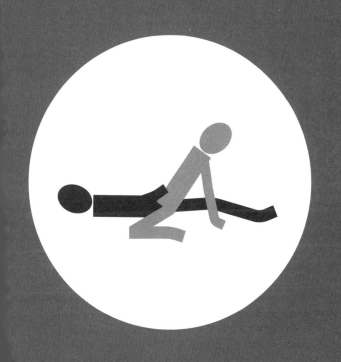

Chapter 4
SEATED POSITIONS

A NATURAL PROGRESSION FROM THE EASIER SUPINE POSITIONS, SEATED POSITIONS CAN GIVE YOU THE CHANCE TO HAVE GREATER CONTACT WITH YOUR PARTNER, DEEPER PENETRATION AND A NEW EXPERIENCE OF EACH OTHER.

The
ROCKING HORSE

INTIMACY: ▼ ▼ ▼ ▼ ▼

SUPPLENESS: ▼ ▼ ▼ ▽ ▽

In this position, the person being penetrated is the active partner.

The passive partner sits cross-legged, perhaps supported by cushions. They can also use their hands for extra support. The active partner then kneels over the passive partner's lap, lowering themselves down until penetration can be achieved. They can hold their partner for support as they use a bouncing or swaying motion to build speed and penetration.

This is a great position for romance, as you can gaze into your partner's eyes throughout.

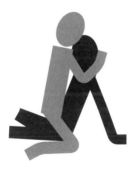

CATHERINE WHEEL

FLEXIBILITY: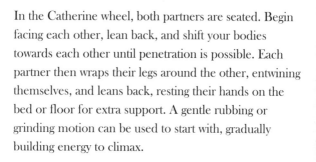

STIMULATION:

In the Catherine wheel, both partners are seated. Begin facing each other, lean back, and shift your bodies towards each other until penetration is possible. Each partner then wraps their legs around the other, entwining themselves, and leans back, resting their hands on the bed or floor for extra support. A gentle rubbing or grinding motion can be used to start with, gradually building energy to climax.

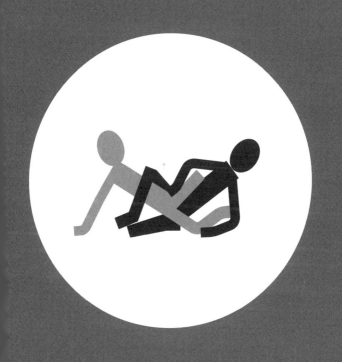

CROUCHING TIGER

DIFFICULTY: ▼ ▼ ▼ ▼ ▼

AGILITY: ▼ ▼ ▼ ▼ ▼

This position takes its name from the crouching position of the passive partner.

The active partner lies on their back at the edge of the bed, with their feet on the floor. The passive partner then squats over the active partner to achieve penetration. Both the movements of the active and passive partners can build momentum in this position, depending on who wants more control. The active partner can hold their partner's bottom if they want more control over movement. During this position, the passive partner's hands are free to give extra pleasure to their partner, or themselves.

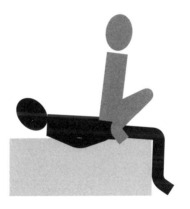

The
FROG

SENSUALITY: ▼ ▼ ▼ ▼ ▽

BALANCE: ▼ ▼ ▼ ▼ ▼

This position is somewhat similar to the crouching tiger, in that the passive partner squats over the active one. In this, however, both partners are sitting, rather than lying down. This allows for a greater sense of closeness and intimacy, letting the passive partner feel held and secure.

The active partner sits at the edge of the bed, leaving room for the passive partner to squat over them. The passive partner lowers themselves down, back to their partner, using their hands to balance, like a frog. Once in this position, the passive partner's bouncing movement or the active partner's thrusting can control the rhythm.

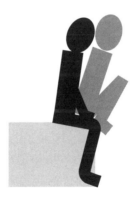

KNEELING CONGRESS

STAMINA: ▼ ▼ ▼ ▽ ▽

CLOSENESS: ▼ ▼ ▼ ▼ ▼

Otherwise known as 'the kneel', this is a great position for romance, as you face each other, so can look into each other's eyes. Additionally, you get full body contact, which allows a greater level of intimacy and romance, as well as heightening sensitivity as different areas of your bodies brush and press together.

To achieve kneeling bliss, the active partner keeps their legs together, while the passive partner straddles them, allowing for penetration. The passive partner can then wrap their arms around the active partner's neck, and move in for a kiss, while the active partner develops a slow, gentle rhythm.

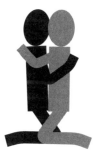

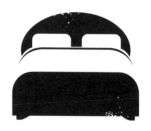

TO HAVE HER HERE IN BED WITH ME, BREATHING ON ME... I COUNT THAT SOMETHING OF A MIRACLE.

HENRY MILLER

Chapter 5

STANDING POSITIONS

PERHAPS MORE ADVENTUROUS,
ESPECIALLY AS THEY TEND TO BE MORE
ENERGETIC AND CAN EASILY BE DONE
OUTSIDE THE BEDROOM, HERE WE LOOK
AT SOME OF THE STANDING POSITIONS
WHICH HAVE BEEN INSPIRED BY THE *KAMA
SUTRA*. THOUGH SOME ARE SUPPORTED,
THESE CAN REQUIRE QUITE A LOT OF
STRENGTH AND STAMINA!

LOVE IS COMPOSED OF A SINGLE SOUL INHABITING TWO BODIES.

ARISTOTLE

The PADLOCK

COMFORT: ▼ ▼ ▽ ▽ ▽

RAUNCHINESS: ▼ ▼ ▼ ▼ ▼

In this position, the active partner is standing while the passive partner sits on top of a piece of furniture, such as a table or kitchen counter, supported by their arms. The active partner stands in front, and the passive partner wraps their legs around them, pulling them in close for deep penetration. The active partner could lean on the surface for balance, or take hold of their partner's bottom to control the speed and depth of penetration.

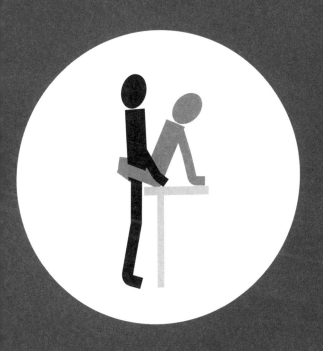

The ASCENT TO DESIRE

EASE: 🖤🖤🤍🤍🤍

WORKOUT LEVEL: 🖤🖤🖤🖤🖤

This could be seen as the 'classic' standing position, and requires at least one partner to be strong, with plenty of stamina.

The active partner stands with their knees slightly bent, making sure they are firmly balanced. The active partner then lifts the passive partner up. The passive partner wraps their legs around the active partner's hips for penetration, and wraps their arms around their partner's

shoulders for closeness and stability. If it helps, the
passive partner can balance their feet on the edge of the
bed or back of the sofa to take some of their own weight.
The downward action of the passive partner's weight
makes this a position for very deep penetration, as well as
being a damn good workout!

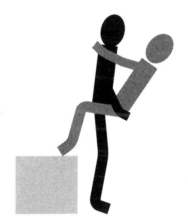

The PLOUGH

FLEXIBILITY: ▼ ▼ ▼ ▼ ▽

CARNALITY: ▼ ▼ ▼ ▼ ▽

Though not strictly a completely upright position, this requires one partner to stand, and to have plenty of stamina.

To achieve the plough position, the passive partner lies at the end of the bed, legs over the edge. The active partner then lifts the passive partner's legs and holds them, either side of their hips, whilst moving in for penetration.

The passive partner needs to support themselves on
their elbows while the active partner holds them up and
controls things from behind – the active partner is fully in
control in this position.

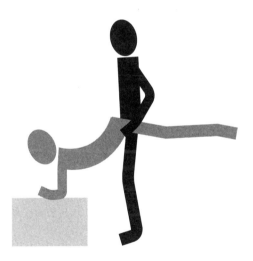

The
LUSTFUL LEG

STRENGTH: ▼ ▼ ▼ ▽ ▽

FLEXIBILITY: ▼ ▼ ▼ ▼ ▼

This is a little more adventurous than the padlock or the ascent to desire, and requires more strength, flexibility and balance, but the result can be great, especially if you enjoy deeper penetration.

Start facing each other. The passive partner should rest one leg on the bed, or another surface, then the active partner can bend down and lift the leg on to their shoulder. The passive partner wraps their arms around

their partner's neck and allows themselves to be pulled
in for penetration. The active partner holds on to their
partner's bottom for extra support and to control
their thrusts.

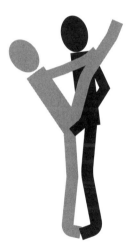

The
CHALLENGE

AGILITY: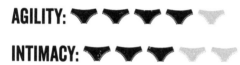

INTIMACY:

This aptly named position is trickier than your average standing position, and requires plenty of leg strength and balance from the passive partner. You'll also need a good, sturdy chair, or something similar.

The passive partner stands on the chair, then bends into a sitting position, elbows on knees. The active partner can then enter from behind, keeping hold of their partner's waist or bottom for added balance and control.

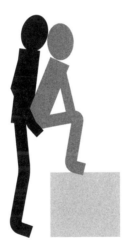

Chapter 6

FOR THE EXTRA-ADVENTUROUS

IF YOU THINK YOU'VE TRIED IT ALL AND
GOT THE T-SHIRT, TRY SOME OF THE MORE
ADVENTUROUS SUGGESTIONS IN THIS
SECTION. THESE ARE NOT FOR THE FAINT-
HEARTED; THEY WILL CHALLENGE YOUR
STAMINA AND, IN SOME CASES,
YOUR BALANCE!

The
EROTIC V

CORE STRENGTH:

SATISFACTION:

This is a challenging seated/standing position, which requires balance. The passive partner rests their bottom at the edge of a table or other firm surface. The active partner stands in front of them, and lets their partner rest a leg against each of their shoulders. The passive partner can wrap their arms around the active partner's neck for extra support. In this position, the active partner enters – this can achieve very deep penetration.

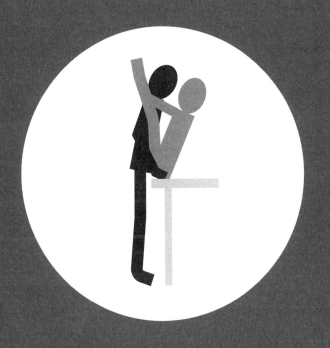

The
APE

LASCIVIOUSNESS: 🩲 🩲 🩲 🩲 🩲

DIFFICULTY: 🩲 🩲 🩲 🩲 🩲

This is an advanced position, and requires strength, stamina, flexibility and balance. For all that it requires, though, it can give intense pleasure as it allows for deep, controlled penetration.

The passive partner lies on their back, and pulls their knees up to their chest. A firm surface such as the floor is better for this position, as it gives better support. The active partner then sits back to allow penetration, resting their back on the passive partner's feet, and controls penetration by moving up and down. They can reach back and hold their partner's wrists for extra support, if needed.

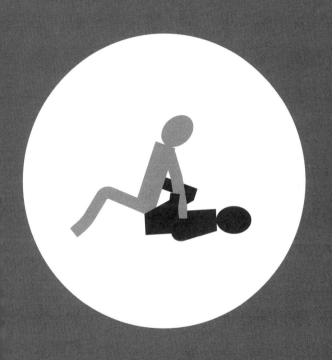

The BRIDGE

SENSUALITY: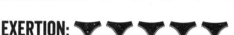

EXERTION:

This one really *is* for the super strong and flexible only!

First, the partner who will be penetrating forms the bridge, by bending over backwards. Then, the passive partner straddles them, lowering themselves down gently to achieve penetration. It is then the penetrated partner who becomes active, using the motion of their legs to control penetration.

It is advised that you don't stay in this position for too long – you wouldn't want to collapse with all that blood rushing to your head!

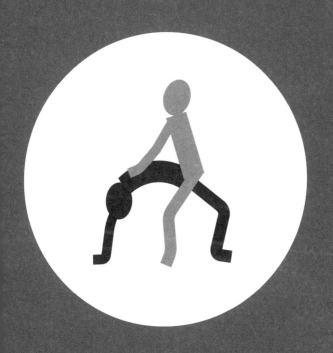

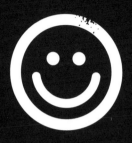

SEX IS ALWAYS ABOUT EMOTIONS. GOOD SEX IS ABOUT FREE EMOTIONS; BAD SEX IS ABOUT BLOCKED EMOTIONS.

DEEPAK CHOPRA

The SUSPENDED SCISSORS

DIFFICULTY: ▼ ▼ ▼ ▼ ▼

STRENGTH: ▼ ▼ ▼ ▼ ▼

BALANCE: ▼ ▼ ▼ ▼ ▼

SEXINESS: ▼ ▼ ▽ ▽ ▽

SATISFACTION: ▼ ▼ ▼ ▽ ▽

FUN: ▼ ▼ ▼ ▼ ▼

This is the most adventurous and the trickiest position we've included in this book! If you want to try something truly athletic, this may be for you.

The passive partner lies on the edge of the bed, with just their calves and feet still supported, with one arm holding themselves up from the floor, while the active partner supports them at the waist.

The active partner then straddles their partner's lower leg, helping hold the upper leg, and penetrates the passive partner while they balance on the edge.

Though this may sound complex, if you have the strength and stamina for it, the natural stimulation from the scissor position, along with the rush of blood to the passive partner's head, can lead to amazing orgasms.

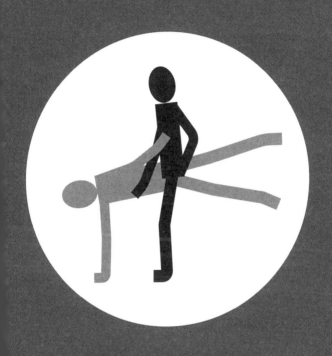

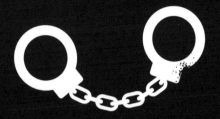

IT IS NOT SEX THAT GIVES THE PLEASURE, BUT THE LOVER.

MARGE PIERCY

Conclusion

We hope you've enjoyed this book, and that it's given you some food for thought! However you choose to use it – as a mini guide or reference book, or just to get your own ideas flowing – we hope that it will help enhance your sex life, and bring you and your partner closer together. Perhaps you will go on to read the original *Kama Sutra* and appreciate the wide knowledge of happy relationships it has continued to impart for centuries.

Checklist

- ☐ **THE BENT KISS**

- ☐ **THE TURNED KISS**

- ☐ **THE KISS THAT KINDLES LOVE**

- ☐ **THE KISS THAT TURNS AWAY**

- ☐ **THE DEMONSTRATIVE KISS**

- ☐ **SOLO FELLATIO**

- ☐ **SOLO CUNNILINGUS**

- ☐ CLASSIC '69'
- ☐ SIDE '69'
- ☐ DOGGY STYLE
- ☐ THE LAP OF LUXURY
- ☐ THE FACE SIT
- ☐ BANDOLEER
- ☐ THE GLOWING TRIANGLE
- ☐ NIRVANA
- ☐ THE SPLITTING BAMBOO

☐ **THE CURLED ANGEL**

☐ **THE CLIP**

☐ **THE ROCKING HORSE**

☐ **CATHERINE WHEEL**

☐ **CROUCHING TIGER**

☐ **THE FROG**

☐ **KNEELING CONGRESS**

☐ **THE PADLOCK**

☐ **THE ASCENT TO DESIRE**

☐ **THE PLOUGH**

☐ **THE LUSTFUL LEG**

☐ **THE CHALLENGE**

☐ **THE EROTIC V**

☐ **THE APE**

☐ **THE BRIDGE**

☐ **THE SUSPENDED SCISSORS**

If you're interested in finding out more about our books, find us on Facebook at **SUMMERSDALE PUBLISHERS** and follow us on Twitter at **@SUMMERSDALE**.

WWW.SUMMERSDALE.COM
